Diabetes:

---

*A Straightforward Step-by-Step
Guide to Naturally Reverse Diabetes Now*

Teresa Fikes

Dedication

Dedicated to my brave husband who struggles with diabetes for his being my test subject on my many recipes that is good for his health.

Table of Contents

Introduction 1

Chapter One 2

What Is Diabetes? 2
   Two Types of Diabetes...2
   Risk Factors for Diabetes: What Increases Your Risk of Diabetes?.................3
   Symptoms of Diabetes...3

Chapter Two 5

Symptoms/consequences of an unhealthy lifestyle 5
   What is a healthy versus an unhealthy diet? 5

Chapter Three 7

Complications of Diabetes...7
   Constraints 7
   Complications 8
   Glaucoma and cataracts 8
   Diabetic ketoacidosis 8
   Digestive problems 8
   Incontinence 8

Chapter Four 9

Foods to eat and why 9
   Great Foods for a diabetic..9
   Tips 12
   Eat Superfoods 12

Chapter Five 15

Foods to avoid 15

Chapter Six..18

Healthy Strategies to Avoid Diabetes 18

Chapter Seven 20

Creating a Diabetic Diet for the Type II Diabetic 20

Carbohydrates 20

Proteins 20

Fats... 21

Bad Fats 22

Dairy Products 23

Whole grains and starchy vegetables.. 24

Starchy vegetables... 24

Starchy vegetables with Plant protein.. 25

Non-Starchy vegetables 26

Fruits 27

Diabetes Superfoods 29

Chapter Eight 30

A Low Carbohydrate Diet for the Type II Diabetic................................. 30

Chapter Nine 32

Exercise- Get up and move! 32

Benefits of Regular Exercise 32

Getting Started with Exercise... 33

Diabetic Complications and Exercise.. 34

Chapter Ten 36

It's all about the lifestyle- once you're free from diabetes STAY free 36

Controlling diabetes to stay free of additional complications.................... 36

Regular Exercise will Keep You Young... 37

Methods to Reduce Stress and Stay Healthy 38

Chapter Eleven 40

Conclusion... 40

About the Author 41

Preview of 'Fermented Foods for Gut Health' 42

Don't forget to check out Teresa's other books on Amazon.com............... 44

Introduction

First of all, I will like to congratulate you on downloading this e-book entitled **Diabetes: A Straightforward Step-by-Step Guide to Naturally Reverse Diabetes Now.**

It is our hope that this book will enable you to learn the basics of the diabetic condition and most importantly how to actively manage your blood sugar levels, and undo the effects of unhealthy lifestyle.

This book takes an insightful look at the basics of a healthy low carbohydrate diet and the ways in which superfoods help you maintain an excellent eating lifestyle.

Other topics covered are the benefits of exercising to a diabetic person and the consequences of a high stress and sedentary lifestyle, which many of us find ourselves in. This book will suggest ways in which you can modify your day-to-day activities so as to undo the negative effects of diabetes and enable you to take hold of your health.

Chapter One

What Is Diabetes?

As a disease of the endocrine system, diabetes affects the body's ability to process sugar in the body. Food eaten is converted into sugar (glucose). Contrary to popular belief, it is not only sweet foods that are converted into sugar in the blood. Carbohydrates and most proteins are also converted into glucose. The pancreas produces insulin, which is used to manage the sugar levels in the blood by carrying sugar to cells that need it. When the pancreas is unable to produce the required amount of insulin or the body is unable to utilize the insulin produced, diabetes occurs.

Two Types of Diabetes

Diabetes is grouped into two distinct types. These are Type I diabetes and Type II diabetes.

Type I diabetes is due to failure of the pancreas. This usually appears in adolescence. Pancreatitis can also lead to type I diabetes in adults. Although type I diabetes cannot be cured, treatment can help manage it. With type I diabetes, the body just cannot produce enough insulin as a result of damaged pancreatic cells. Also called insulin dependent diabetes mellitus (IDDM) or juvenile diabetes, it affects about a tenth (10 percent) of all diabetics.

Type II diabetes is as a result of poor eating habits, insulin resistance, unhealthy lifestyle, and obesity. This condition can be reversed. Adults usually develop type II diabetes when the body cannot effectively utilize insulin produced by the pancreas. Also called non-insulin dependent diabetes mellitus or adult-onset diabetes, it affects about nine-tenth (90 percent) of all diabetics.

This book covers type II diabetes.

Risk Factors for Diabetes: What Increases Your Risk of Diabetes?

- Being obese or being overweight.

- Over 45 and overweight.

- Having a family history of diabetes.

- Having gestational diabetes in the past.

- Suffering from impaired glucose tolerance.

- Suffering from insulin resistance.

- Suffering from polycystic ovary syndrome.

- Living a sedentary lifestyle.

- Ethnic background - Hispanic/Latino Americans, African-Americans, Alaska natives Asian-Americans, Native Americans, and Pacific Islanders, are more likely to suffer from type II diabetes

Symptoms of Diabetes

- Dark patches on the skin

- Dry mouth and itchy skin.

- Hearing loss

- Heavy snoring

- Hunger and fatigue.

- Nausea, vomiting or stomach pain

- Peeing more often and being thirstier.

- Sweet smelling urine

- Tingling in the hands or feet

- Unexplained weight loss

- Blurred vision.

- Changes in your eyesight

- Yeast infections.

- Slow-healing sores or cuts.

- Pain or numbness in your feet or legs

Chapter Two

Symptoms/consequences of
an unhealthy lifestyle

Unhealthy lifestyle is one of the main causes of type II diabetes. A sedentary lifestyle, lack of exercise, unhealthy diet, and high-stress levels all add to result in an unhealthy lifestyle.

What is a healthy versus an unhealthy diet?

It is imperative that you are able to define what a healthy diet is - a healthy diet is one that has the recommended proportions and amounts of protein, fats, carbohydrates, minerals, and vitamins. An unhealthy diet, on the other hand, does not have the needed proteins, good fat, carbohydrates, minerals, and vitamins in the recommended proportions and amounts. Unhealthy diets are as a result of by the under-consumption of needed nutrients, and the overconsumption of salt, sugar cholesterol, saturated fats, and trans fats. As a result, the outcome of an unhealthy diet is malnutrition, obesity, and/or weight gain.

While a healthy diet improves the immune system, reduces your risk of chronic illness, and diseases, an unhealthy diet can cause osteoporosis, cancer, obesity, diabetes, cardiovascular diseases, and many others.

As defined by the Centers for Disease Control and Prevention (CDC), being overweight means having a BMI (body mass index) of above 25. Few portions of whole grains, vegetables, and fruits and too many portions of meats, fried foods, and fatty foods often result in a poor diet which in turn leads to overweight and obesity. Another cause of obesity is the high intake of carbonated sugary drinks. These sweet beverages can have as much as 9.5 teaspoons for every 12 fluid ounces, which is very high. A sedentary lifestyle coupled with lack of proper exercise does not help either.

Furthermore, being obese means having a BMI (body mass index) of 30 and above. Having a body mass index of 35 and more is classified as morbidly obese. Diabetes is not the only contribution of obesity. Obesity also increases the risk of stroke, erectile dysfunction in men, infertility in women, osteoarthritis, sleep apnea, high levels of bad cholesterol, high blood pressure, certain cancers, type II diabetes, heart diseases, gallbladder disease, and liver disease.

Chapter Three

Complications of Diabetes

Once a person becomes a diabetic as an adult, a lifestyle change happens. A diabetic has to watch every calorie they consume, so they can adjust their insulin intake.

If the diabetic is not yet on insulin, there will be pills to take and blood sugar to measure every day. There will be quarterly doctor visits for a hemoglobin A1C test, which may not have been necessary before. There are some jobs that are proBeing diagnosed with diabetes comes with many lifestyle changes. Since a diabetic needs to adjust his or her insulin intake, they need to keep track of every calorie. High blood sugar, which is termed as hyperglycemia, affects several diabetic patients, especially those who do not actively manage their blood sugar level. This condition can lead to several complications.

Constraints

For a diabetic who is not on insulin, there are pills that you need to take in addition to recording your blood sugar levels every morning. In addition, there need to do a hemoglobin A1C test every 3 months. Furthermore, being diabetic prohibits you from doing some activities, for example in the United States, diabetics are not qualified to carry a driver's license.

Complications

It is important that you monitor your diabetes, as morning blood sugar levels above 100 can lead to conditions such as kidney damage, heart attack, stroke, blindness and nerve damage to the hands and legs. Poor circulation and nerve damage coupled can even result in limb amputation.

Glaucoma and cataracts

Other signs of diabetic uncontrolled blood sugar are cataracts and glaucoma. Glaucoma, when left untreated, can easily lead to blindness. In the same vein, diabetic retinopathy, which is also caused by high blood sugar, can also lead to blindness.

Diabetic ketoacidosis

Having a high blood sugar level can cause diabetic to go into diabetic ketoacidosis. This can result in a coma and even death.

Digestive problems

Another complication that can arise when blood sugar levels is not checked, digestive problems such as Gastroparesis are a result of damaged nerves in the stomach, which is directly caused by high blood sugars. As such, food ingested digests slowly. This makes the individual prone to stomach cancers and blockages.

Incontinence

Other complications, such as elimination, can occur. Since the nerves in the sphincter and bladder can become numb, a diabetic can become incontinent as the disease progresses. As such, the diabetic patient may not feel the urge to use the bathroom until the periodic elimination of urine has begun.

Chapter Four

Foods to eat and why

Once food is eaten, it is converted to sugar, which is then burnt for energy. For a diabetic, this sugar is immediately converted into fat and stored.

Foods with high glycemic index take short time to convert into fat; on the other hand, foods such as simple carbohydrates are quickly converted. It essential that diabetics avoid simple carbohydrates, such as white bread, sugar, and rice. These are turned into sugar much quicker.

Complex carbohydrates such as brown rice, whole grains, and vegetables and fruits have a high fiber base and as such takes much longer to digest. The fiber helps fight colon cancer and the slower digestion is also preferable.

Great Foods for a diabetic

Almond is a great source of protein and curbs hunger. It is also a food known for decreasing blood sugar levels. It also has heart health benefits. Low in carbohydrates and high in magnesium, this is a great snack to help you maintain low blood sugar levels.

Beet is another superfood that has to be on every diabetic's menu. This vegetable is high in metabolites, folate, potassium, and importantly fiber. Metabolites are molecules that aid in cellular functions. They aid in increasing liver function and lowering insulin resistance and are beneficial to cardiovascular health.

Celery is a great source of molybdenum, and potassium, vitamins A and C, folate, and vitamin K. the vitamin K in celery helps prevent H. pylori bacteria. Studies have shown there is a strong link between high blood glucose levels/diabetes and H. pylori bacteria.

Cinnamon's health benefits are well known. Adding flavor to buns and other foods is not the only thing it is good for. It is great for stabilizing blood sugar. A cup of cinnamon tea is an excellent way to reduce sugar craving.

Dark leafy greens, spinach, and broccoli are also healthy choices. They have tons of minerals, vitamins, and fiber. Low in carbohydrates and calories, you can consume more without taking in many calories. We recommend that half your plate should be greens.

Fishes such as halibut, mackerel, herring, tuna, and salmon are high in omega 3 fatty acids, which is healthy and great for the heart. They are also a great source of protein and low in calories. These foods will ensure you maintain a good blood sugar level and also helps reduce LDL cholesterol. Reduction in red meat also helps reduce LDL cholesterol. Another great way to reduce cholesterol and triglycerides is through consumption of high fiber foods.

Garlic and garlic oil is also good for a diabetic since it is good for the heart. You should try to include garlic in your diet since it helps reduce blood sugar when it stimulates the body to produce and use insulin efficiently.

Oatmeal is a healthy food that should be on every diabetic's diet. It is full of fiber as such takes long to digest, and it is full of energy. It will have you sated for longer.

Quinoa is one of the best foods you can have in your diet as a diabetic. It is high in fiber, protein, vitamins, and minerals. It has a low glycemic index and tastes great.

When taken with cheese before bed, apple cider vinegar can lower blood glucose by as much as 6 percent. One oz. of cheese and two tablespoons of apple cider vinegar before bed is all you need to stop the Somogyi phenomenon, and thus reduce blood sugar levels first thing the next morning.

WARNING: It is important to discuss vinegar consumption with your doctor if you have gastroparesis.

Recap: High fiber foods are more beneficial to a diabetic and are also more nutritious as compared to simple carbohydrates and sugar.

Here are some foods in include in your diet.

- Barley
- Beans
- Berries
- Dairy
- Dark chocolate
- Dates
- Flaxseed
- Greens
- Lentils

- Oats

- Peanut butter

- Salmon

- Tuna

- Walnuts

Tips

- It is important that a diabetic patient eat enough protein, low amounts of carbohydrates, and a lot of fibrous vegetables. Cinnamon and garlic are also great additions since they allow for effective use of insulin by the body.

- Drinking a lot of water is good for you, as much as an ounce per pound of your body weight on a day-to-day basis.

- You can substitute some foods for healthier choices. Instead of processed cereal, eat steel cut oats for breakfast. Instead of fruit juice or fruit leather, eat whole fruits. Instead of fried potatoes, eat baked potato chips. Instead of light-colored veggies, eat dark leafy greens. Instead of processed carbohydrates, eat whole grains

Eat Superfoods

High in vitamins and minerals, polyphenols, and antioxidants, superfoods help your body fight viruses, illness, and free radicals. It is important that you add superfoods to your diet. They will have you feeling and performing better.

- Black beans have full fiber and iron content in addition to antioxidants.

- Blueberries are high in phytonutrients, which helps prevent cancer by slowing down the effects of free radicals. It also improves cognitive functions.

- Broccoli is full of vitamin C.

- Dark chocolate is great as it helps with depression, improves the immune system, improves blood circulation, and reduces blood pressure. Dark chocolate is at least 70 percent cacao.

- Kale is high in phytonutrients, it helps prevent ovarian and breast cancers and other cancers by slowing down the effects of free radicals. It also improves cognitive functions.

- Oat is full of magnesium and high fiber content and helps maintain a healthy blood glucose level, prevent colon cancer, and reduce bad cholesterol.

- Pistachios are also high fiber nuts that improve good cholesterol levels and reduce bad cholesterol levels.

- Pumpkins are full of potassium and beta-carotene. Frequent intake improves eye health and reduces blood pressure.

- Red bell pepper is high in vitamin C (about twice as much as an orange), lycopene, and beta-carotene - all of which are important for a healthy eye.

- Salmon and Sardines are both full of omega 3 fatty acids. These beneficial fatty acids help increase HDL/good cholesterol and reduce LDL/ bad cholesterol, inflammation, and risk of cardiovascular diseases. Sardines also come in cans already cooked.

- Spinach is high in phytonutrients and just a cup contains double the recommended daily requirements of vitamin K. it helps prevent macular degeneration.

- Tomatoes are high in lycopene, which helps prevent cancer by protecting you from harmful UV light produced by the sun.

Chapter Five

Foods to avoid

As a diabetic, there are several foods you need to avoid, foods that are a part of American culture. The high levels of processed carbohydrates, sugar, fat and bad cholesterol make these foods harmful to a person with diabetes.

- Store bought pie
- Store bought cookies/biscuits
- Store bought cake
- Restaurant/fast food outlet burgers
- Processed lunchmeats
- Processed hot dogs
- Pastries
- Nachos
- Fruit smoothies
- Fruit juice beverages
- Pizza
- Frozen Entrees
- Fried battered chicken
- French fries
- Flavored water
- Battered fish and greasy fries

- Fast food outlet milkshakes
- Fast food
- Doughnuts
- Deep-fried Chinese foods such as sesame chicken
- Coffee drinks such as Frappuccino and cappuccino (black coffee with no cream and no sweeteners is good though)
- Cinnamon rolls with icing
- Carbonated drinks
- Buttered biscuits and sausage gravy

The above foods are high in calories, transfats, fats, sugar, and salt, making them harmful to a diabetic. They spike up blood glucose levels and are a nightmare.

As a diabetic, there are also some regular foods you should avoid. Some fruits such as watermelons and bananas may not be obvious choices, but they should be avoided as well.

- White foods such as white sugar, white salt, white rice, white gravy, white flour, and white bread
- Alcohol
- Bananas
- Watermelons
- Breakfast pastries such as pop tarts
- Chinese foods
- Dried fruits
- Fatty meat
- Fried foods
- Fruit juices

- Full-fat dairy foods
- High carbohydrate energy bars
- Pasta with Alfredo sauce
- Prepackaged baked goods
- Prepackaged snacks
- Pre-sweetened cereal such Fruit Loops
- Smoked Meats
- Sweet foods
- Trail mix

Chapter Six

Healthy Strategies to Avoid Diabetes

Even if you are not diabetic but you have a sneaky feeling you may be a prime candidate for this condition, here are some strategies to help you prevent type II diabetes,

1. A thirty-minute work daily is a great way to reduce the risk of diabetes by as much as 40 percent. This is because walking upsurges insulin receptors in cells. When there is much fat stored in the body, it inhibits insulin receptors. Exercise removes this fat from outside the cell, thus helping the receptors to function efficiently.

2. Between lunch and supper, snack on salads with vinegar-based dressing daily. While the vinegar helps with the efficient use of insulin, salad reduces appetite and increases fiber intake.

3. Cinnamon is great for reducing blood glucose levels. Just 3 capsules of cinnamon a day for 3 months can lower blood sugar levels by as much as a tenth (10 percent), according to a study.

4. Do not take fast food. Even occasional consumption is dangerous. Eating fast food just twice a day can increase insulin resistance by 200 percent.

5. Drinking coffee with no sweeteners and no creamers is a healthy choice as far as you do not overdo it. Green tea

also works fine. The caffeine and antioxidants in these beverages help increase metabolism and sugar absorption.

6. Frequent consumption of red meat increases your risks of developing diabetes. Studies show that women who eat red meat five times in a week are almost 30 percent times likelier to become diabetic.

7. High fiber cereals are better than pre-sweetened cereal. Even cereals such as cornflakes are not advisable. Stick to high fiber cereals such as oatmeal and bran cereals.

8. If you are overweight, try losing weight. Even a small amount of weight loss such as 10 percent of your weight can reduce the risk of diabetes by as much as 50 percent.

9. Living alone also increases your chances of developing diabetes by as much as 2.5 times in women. Get involved in social activities.

10. Stress is a huge determinant of high blood sugar. It is important to cut down on stress. Find ways to do that.

11. Try to get a lot of sleep. Men who sleep six hours or less a night increase the risk of diabetes by as much as 200 percent while persons who have eight hours or more of sleep a night reduced their risk of diabetes by three times.

12. Regular blood tests are the surest way to know your blood sugar level. If it is determined that you are pre-diabetic early you can actively work on preventing it.

Chapter Seven

Creating a Diabetic Diet for the Type II Diabetic

As a type II diabetic, you need to eat specifically to cater for your condition. Knowing what fats, carbohydrates, and proteins are, and the amounts in which to consume them is essential.

Carbohydrates

Carbohydrates are a great energy source. Basically, we have 3 carbohydrates, namely - sugar, starch, and fiber.

The body needs carbohydrate to function, so you cannot just stop eating it. However, limiting the amount eaten is essential. As a diabetic, you will want to limit carbohydrate portions to 45 grams per meal and 15 grams per snack. It is important to check the nutritional value found on the label of the food. That way you know just how much you are taking it. If there is no nutritional label, knowing the weight of the food can help you determine just how much carbohydrate is in it via a quick internet search.

Bread, dried beans, fruits, grains, rice, starchy vegetables like carrots and vegetables are examples of carbohydrates.

Proteins

Proteins are often referred to as the building blocks of the body as they provide essential amino acids needed for muscle development. Proteins include animal protein such as beef, eggs, fish, milk, pork, poultry, and seafood, while some plant proteins include soy nuts and edamame, hummus and falafel, nuts like peanut and almond, and tempeh and tofu.

With the exceptions of lentils and dried beans, protein does not increase blood glucose level and does not have carbohydrates.

Include protein in every meal and even as a bedtime snack. 2-5 ounces of protein per serving is recommended depending on kidney function and diet plan. Since diabetics can develop kidney disease due to hyperglycemia, which damages the blood vessels, therefore a serving of 2 ounces may be best for those who suffer kidney diseases.

Fats

Fats can be good fat or bad fat. Diabetics should limit fats to 20 grams a day. Just a slice of cheese has as much as 8 grams of fat, so you can eat very little fat.

Polyunsaturated Fats - These are healthy fats, examples include

- Safflower oil
- Salad dressing
- Sunflower oil

Omega 3 fatty acids reduce bad cholesterol and triglycerides and lower the risks of heart attacks and strokes. As such, omega 3 fatty acids are good fats. Examples include

- Herrin
- Mackerel
- Salmon
- Sardines
- Tuna
- Flaxseed oil and flaxseed

- Tofu and soy foods

Some other sources of good fats include

- Avocado
- Canola oil
- Nuts
- Olive oil
- Olives
- Peanut butter
- Peanut oil
- Sesame oil
- Sunflower oil

Bad Fats

These saturated fats should be avoided as they spike triglyceride, cholesterol, and blood sugar levels. Trans fats are another type of fat you should seek to avoid at all times. Example of trans fat is shortening melted to make cooking oil. Trans fats are gotten from melted fat. When they get into the blood arteries, they coagulate and stick to artery walls. They eventual get free of artery walls make their way through the circulatory system and end up lodging in the heart. This leads to heart attacks.

Some sources of bad fats include

- 2% milk
- Cream sauce
- Bacon
- Bologna
- Butter

- Coconut oil
- Cracklings
- Fatback
- Full fat cheese
- Gravy prepared with meat grease
- Ground beef
- Hot dogs
- Hydrogenated oils
- Ice cream
- Italian sausage
- Lard
- Margarine
- Milk chocolate
- Movie theatre butter
- Palm kernel oil
- Polish sausage
- Salt pork
- Sausage
- Spareribs
- Whole milk

Dairy Products

These are several dairy products on the market. With milk, there is nonfat/skimmed milk, 2%, and full cream or whole milk. Nonfat is best for a diabetic. A serving of nonfat yogurt has 6 grams protein and 12 grams carbohydrates. It is the same with a cup of nonfat milk. Greek yogurt is a healthier alternative since it has more protein content and lowers carbohydrate content.

Milk has a low glycemic index, is full of calcium, and helps reduce belly fat.

Whole grains and starchy vegetables

Whole grain has high fiber content, making them the healthy choice. Whole grain foods usually have whole grains written on the label. Read the ingredients to make sure. Whole grain foods should not include sugar, sweeteners, and corn syrup and must have a high percentage of whole grain as an ingredient.

Some fantastic whole grain foods are

- Brown rice
- Buckwheat
- Buckwheat flour
- Cornmeal
- Millet
- Popcorn
- Quinoa
- Sorghum
- Whole grain barley
- Whole oats
- Whole-wheat flour
- Wild rice

Starchy vegetables

Starchy vegetables are needed since they contain fiber, vitamins, and minerals your body needs. As usual, watch the carbohydrate content. Half a cup of starchy carbohydrate is equivalent to 15 grams of carbohydrates with the exception of acorn squash and pumpkin, which have less carbohydrate (7.5 grams per half a cup). White rice also has 15 grams of carbohydrates per half a cup.

Some starchy vegetables

- Butternut or acorn squash
- Corn
- English peas or snap peas
- Potato
- Pumpkin

Starchy vegetables with Plant protein

While foods that are a good source of plant protein usually contain carbohydrates, they also contain much protein. Choose a day out of the week when you eat no meat to lower red meat consumption.

Some sources of plant protein

- Black-eyed peas
- Butter peas
- Dried beans, like pinto, navy, and Lima
- Lentils,
- Refried beans (fat-free)
- Split peas
- Vegetarian baked beans.

Non-Starchy vegetables

Containing phytonutrients, fiber, vitamins and minerals, non-starchy vegetables are good for you and as such, you should consume about 5 servings a day.

The following vegetables contain little to no carbohydrates so are great for sating your hunger without adding extra calories or spiking your blood sugar.

- Turnips
- Tomato
- Salad lettuce, leaf, butter, chicory, parsley, red leaf, watercress, romaine, spinach
- Onions
- Okra
- Mushrooms
- Leeks
- Kohlrabi
- Jicama
- Hearts of palm
- Greens, turnip, mustard, collard, kale
- Cucumber
- Coleslaw prepared with vinegar dressing
- Celery
- Cauliflower
- Carrots
- Cactus
- Cabbage, green, Chinese, purple, book Choy

- Brussels sprouts
- Beets
- Beans (fresh green)
- Bean sprouts
- Bamboo shoots
- Baby corn
- Asparagus
- Arugula
- Artichokes

Fruits

Fruits are a great source of minerals, vitamins, and fiber. Processed fruits such as canned fruits and dried fruits may contain added sugar.

A small fruit has 15 grams of carbohydrates and qualifies as a serving.

2 tablespoons of dried fruits have 15 grams of carbohydrates. Similarly, sweetened cranberries, dried cherries, dates, and raisins are 2 tablespoons per serving. However, cup of fresh berries including frozen fresh berries is one serving.

Fresh fruit foods can include

- Strawberries
- Raspberries
- Plums
- Pears
- Peaches
- Oranges

- Nectarines
- Loganberries
- Limes
- Lemons
- Kiwi
- Huckleberries
- Grapefruit
- Fruit cocktail
- Figs
- Cherries
- Cantaloupe
- Blueberries
- Blackberries
- Bananas
- Apricots
- Apples

Knowing the glycemic index of foods will better help you determine if a food is suitable for you. Low glycemic index foods are better for a diabetic as they do not spike blood sugar levels as quickly as high glycemic index foods. Examples of low glycemic index foods are oatmeal, beans, peas, vegetables, Fruits, and whole grains; while examples of high glycemic index foods include white bread, soft drinks, fruit juice drinks, cakes, and doughnuts.

A meal should include 50% green vegetables, 25% lean proteins (boiled, grilled, broiled or baked, never fried), and 25%

carbohydrates. Fried foods should be avoided at all cost and should be eaten rarely if you must.

It is important to eat 3 meals and snack 2-3 times a day. A bedtime snack will ensure your blood sugar level does not fluctuate wildly.

Diabetes Superfoods

These foods should be included in your diets since they are high in phytonutrients, minerals, vitamins, fiber, calcium, and antioxidants. You should count the portions so you ensure you are eating right. These foods also have a low glycemic index.

- Walnuts
- Sweet potatoes
- Oatmeal
- Flaxseed
- Fish high in Omega-3 fatty acids
- Nonfat yogurt
- Nonfat milk
- Dried beans
- Dark, leafy vegetables
- Citrus fruits
- Barley

Remember that 1 serving of carbohydrates is 15 grams of carbohydrates.

Chapter Eight

A Low Carbohydrate Diet for the Type II Diabetic

Keeping track of your carbohydrate intake is one of the most effective and easiest diet plans for a diabetic if you wish to maintain a controlled blood glucose level. When carbohydrate is kept low, blood sugar reduces. It also allows you to feel more energetic and less hungry at the same time.

However, before you try out a low carbohydrate diet, you need to consult with your doctor. This way you and your doctor can decide portions that are healthy for your liver and kidney.

According to ADA (American Diabetic Association), the recommended intake of carbohydrates should be 180 grams for a regular diabetic diet. While some patients can maintain a controlled blood sugar level with this amount of carbohydrate, many cannot. As such, they need to reduce the amount of carbohydrate eaten. Depending on your weight and height, you can decide on the right amount with your doctor.

However, following the recommended ADA amount, you can have

- 3 servings of carbohydrates for breakfast,

- 1 serving of carbohydrates for midmorning snack,

- 3 servings of carbohydrates for lunch,

- 1 serving of carbohydrates for midafternoon snack,

- 3 servings of carbohydrates for supper

- 1 serving as bedtime snack.

* 1 serving = 15 grams of carbohydrate

Since this amount is excessively much for many, a low carbohydrate diet may yield better weight results. I recommend a 6 serving diet plan, which is a total of 90 carbohydrates daily.

- 2 servings of carbohydrates for breakfast,

- No or negligible amount of carbohydrates in your midmorning snack,

- 1 servings of carbohydrates for lunch,

- No or negligible amount of carbohydrates in midafternoon snack,

- 2 servings of carbohydrates for supper

- 1 serving as bedtime snack

The midafternoon and midmorning snacks should be proteins and vegetables with no carbohydrates such as celery, and other dark leafy greens. Drink a lot of water more than 64 ounces, and eat a lot of salads (with no carbohydrates) in other to avoid constipation.

Chapter Nine

Exercise- Get up and move!

As a diabetic, exercise is crucial. You need to get the blood flowing and lower blood sugar. A 30-minute stroll can reduce blood sugar by 50 points.

When exercising, your blood sugar level needs to be above 100. Test to ensure this and get some carbohydrates, if the blood sugar level is below 100.

Benefits of Regular Exercise

Exercise has to be an integral part of a diabetic's life and therapy. I recommended 30 minutes of exercise a day. You can divide this into three 10-minute walks, or two 15-minute walks or a single 30-minute walk. Here are some reasons to exercise.

1. Exercise allows cells to receive and efficiently use insulin when previously they could not.

2. Exercise allows cells to use insulin over 24 hours after the exercise.

3. Exercise enables dormant cells use insulin already available.

4. Exercise reduces blood sugar levels.

5. Exercise stimulates muscles to use insulin.

Hypoglycemia is a condition that many diabetics face. This condition occurs when blood glucose levels fall below 70. This should be treated straight away. Take these steps to ensure your blood glucose level is above 70.

1. Test blood glucose level.

2. Consume a serving of carbohydrates (15 grams) and a serving of protein.

3. Wait 15 minutes and test blood glucose level.

4. If blood glucose is still below 70 points, repeat the step 2 and 3.

5. Ensure your exercise and food intake is adjusted accordingly.

Getting Started with Exercise

It is not a good to get up one day and start exercising vigorously, if you have not exercised in a while. Start gradually. Follow these guidelines for a successful exercise session.

- Start with 5 minutes of warm up such as stretching. Then you do a 5-minute cool down. Stretching is applicable in this situation as well.

- Dizziness, chest pain, and breathlessness are not positive signs. If any occurs, stop exercising immediately. If the pain continues after you have stopped exercising, see your doctor or visit the emergency room immediately

- Exercise should not be strenuous. Use the talk test to determine this. If you able to talk during a workout, then it is the right level of exercise. If not, then take the exercise down a notch.

- Have an exercise partner. If you cannot find a partner, you should at least ensure you have a medic alert bracelet on and cellular phone in case of an emergency.

- If blood glucose level drops below 70, test and adjust it as needed.

- In uncomfortable temperatures too hot or too cold, exercise indoors since a diabetic heart finds it difficult adjusting to extreme temperatures. The indoors provide a better-regulated temperature condition.

- When you are diabetic, even small cuts and wounds can be problematical. Check your feet for blisters, bruising and any other injury every day. Wear clean socks, and footwear designed for exercising (not dress shoes).

Diabetic Complications and Exercise

As a diabetic, there are complications such as kidney disease, heart disease, peripheral vascular disease, neuropathy, high blood pressure, or retinopathy, which have to be accounted for when exercising. To be safe, exercise 10 minutes at a time. The workout schedule should be three 10-minute sessions with 5-minute rest sessions in-between.

Do a different exercise each 10-minute session. A full workout should include all muscle groups.

- Chair exercises

- Cycling with recumbent bicycles

- Fishing

- Gardening

- Nu-wave or recumbent exercise machine

- Walking

- Water exercises

- Working with light weights, consult with doctor first

Chapter Ten

It's all about the lifestyle- once you're free from diabetes STAY free

Diabetes cannot be cured; however, it can be reversed or controlled. Once your diabetes is controlled, you need to ensure it stays that way. Here are some things to do to control your diabetes.

Controlling diabetes to stay free of additional complications

1. Be active. Do not remain seated for long periods. Go for additional walks besides your exercise routine. Walk more and do a physical activity once a week with a friend. Have a hobby such as water sports, tennis, fishing, or bowling. Do an activity that does not involve sitting and eating that you enjoy and involves much movement. Just be active.

2. Drink 8 or more glasses of water a day.

3. Eat 160 or fewer grams of carbohydrates a day. Ensure your diet is as healthy as it can be.

4. Get your hemoglobin A1C tested every 3 months.

5. Keep blood glucose level in check. Test your blood glucose every 2 days just to ensure it is in a safe range.

6. Reduce stress levels through meditation, gardening, and other ways.

7. Sleep at least 8 hours each night.

8. Work out 30 minutes 5 days in a week.

Regular Exercise will Keep You Young

The benefits of exercising as a diabetic have been covered. What of the benefits of exercising in general? Exercises can keep you young, and here is how.

1. As you age, your balance deteriorates and your risk of falling increases. Regular movement will improve your balance. When you spend more of your day sedentary, your risk of falls doubles as you lose muscle dexterity and strength. Frequent exercise keeps muscles strong, dexterous, and flexible.

2. Exercise enables you to increase metabolism rate, which helps you, maintain a good weight as your body burns calories.

3. Exercise keeps you flexible. Lack of exercise results in achy and stiff muscles reduced muscle control and bad balance.

4. Exercising reduces osteoporosis since bone loses strength, as you grow old. Exercise strengthens the bones.

5. Keep your energy levels up through frequent exercises, which in turn allows you to do volunteer work. Consecutively this will improve your emotional state, lower depression, and improve self-esteem. You also give back to society.

6. Working out at the gym or frequenting an exercise class improves social skills as you meet people. This is important since as we grow, we need to adapt our social skills to keep up with new social groups. With age comes a

loss of friends as some relocate, get ill, form new social circles, or even pass away.

Methods to Reduce Stress and Stay Healthy

To stay healthy it is important that you reduce stress. There are several activities that can help you de-stress and relax. Here are some suggestions.

- Practice breathing exercises

- Get involved in a hobby such as bowling or gardening.

- Get a professional massage with scented oils.

- Go for a walk with your dog and spend time with her.

- Do guided visualization - this is a great relaxation activity.

- Drink hot tea with cinnamon and honey or maple syrup - this is a great way to relax.

- Hug a loved one for 10 or more seconds.

- Meditate - just a few minutes daily will help improve memory and cognitive functions. Lighting scented candles can help with meditating.

- Listen to relaxing music from classical to rock and roll; choose a genre you enjoy.

- Do Progressive muscle relaxation exercises - start out by tensing and relaxing the toes the move up until you get to the neck and head.

- See a therapist. The therapist can help you de-stress.

- Self-hypnosis is also an effective relaxation tool.

- Spend time with a friend.

- Start a garden or an art project.

- Take a dance class.

- Take a siesta during the day.

- Take walks in the park.

- Watch a comedy - this can be very relaxing.

- Take up yoga - both floor yoga, and chair yoga are beneficial.

Chapter Eleven

Conclusion

I will like to once again thank you for downing this e-book entitled **Diabetes: A Straightforward Step-by-Step Guide to Naturally Reverse Diabetes Now.**

It is my expectation that this book will enable you to manage your diabetes through exercise and healthy eating.

The final step is to adopt a healthy lifestyle, which includes eating well, exercising, and reducing stress.

As a final point, if this book has been of help to you and you enjoyed it, kindly review it and share your thoughts on Amazon. Your reviews are greatly welcomed.

Cheers and all the best on your journey.

About the Author

Teresa has over 40 years of homesteading experience. She loves anything to do with living off the land on and off the grid. She believes in being self-sufficient. She raises her own foods, medicines, and crafts. Also, she is a really big fan of clean eating and pressure cooker recipes, as you can see within many of her different Homesteading series of books and e-books. Teresa specializes in and is a fan of Homesteading Skills which include raising meat rabbits, chickens, goats, hogs, cows, horses, ducks, poultry, and dogs, as well has all kinds of fruits, vegetables and herbs. She collects wild foods and hunts for what she doesn't raise on her small farm.

Teresa's homesteading series includes many book topics such as Home Brewing, slow cooker, clean eating, instant pot, crock pot, electric pressure cooker recipes, baking recipes, preserving, foraging, planting, building, and the list goes on.

Having a well-stocked pantry of easy to open and serve jars of food is essential for a busy family, whether farming, survival prepping, or just the normal city dweller. Follow Teresa to discover more about Homesteading Life Skills.

More about the Arden Marketing Enterprises at: Arden-ent.com

Preview of
'Fermented Foods for Gut Health'

Discover the beneficial techniques of fermentation for a healthier gut!

In Fermented Foods for Gut Health, we will take you through the simple fermentation process, its benefits to your body.

With the scare of not using some form of antibacterial soap, sanitizers or pasteurized foods and dairy products, we are killing off not only the bad bacteria which is harmful to our bodies, but the good bacteria that is to our bodies for attaining optimum health too. It is a trend today to pay for expensive probiotic pills on eating huge amounts of yogurt to replace the good bacteria that are destroyed.

Many of the benefits include:

- Protects against pathogenic bacteria

- Improves digestion

- Helps your body to more effectively absorb nutrients from food

- Fermentation is a natural and safe method of food preservation, and doesn't involve any chemicals or artificial ingredients

- Not to mention it is easy and inexpensive to do

As the bacteria and yeast feed on sugars surrounding it, enzymes are released to break down the large food particles. In other words, fermented foods are predigested and it is full of enzymes, which the body needs.

Fermenting food is not a new concept. It has been around for thousands of years. Something that has been around that long has something to say about health. This is not just a way of preserving foods but also a way of eating healthier and having a healthier life.

Fermented Foods for Gut Health book will show you how to save some money while enjoying delicious ways to improve the gut flora for a better digestive system.

Click here to check out the rest of (Fermented Foods for Gut Health) on Amazon.

Don't forget to check out Teresa's other books on Amazon.com.

Below you'll find some of my other books that are popular on Amazon and Kindle as well. Simply click on the links below to check them out. Alternatively, you can visit my author page on Amazon to see other work done by me.

Alkaline Diet Lifestyle: De-Alkaline Your Body for a Healthier Life

Fermented Foods for Gut Health: How Kimchi and Sauerkraut Can Improve Your Gut Health

Make Your Own Honey Mead at Home: The Homestead Series (Volume 2)

Brew Your Own Beer

The Burn Everything Cookbook: Stories and Recipe of Lean Times

Spirit Guides: Work and Bond with your Spirit Guide

How to Build a Moonshine Still plus recipes

If the links do not work, for whatever reason, you can simply search for these titles on the Amazon website to find them. Or try my Author page

Coming Soon

From my Homestead Series:

How to Make Bannock Bread

It's Only Gravy! 30 Delicious Recipes

Did Someone Say Fresh Beer?: Homebrewed Beers

How to Can Stews and Soups